LIGHTEN UP

29 Playful Lessons

TO HELP YOU LEARN THE

ALEXANDER TECHNIQUE

MARK JOSEFSBERG

Edited by Jessica Penzias

Drawings by Ricky Castillo

LIGHTEN UP

29 Playful Lessons to Help You Learn the Alexander Technique

Edited by Jessica Penzias.
Drawings by Ricky Castillo.

ISBN: 979-8-35091-643-0

CONTENTS

PREFACE

I slumped home with my first school trumpet when I was ten years old. It was dented, tarnished, and smelled like fish, but I cleaned it up and loved playing it right from the start.

And right from the start, I played with my trumpet pointed down—because *I* was pointed down. My neck poked forward and down, and my shoulders rounded downward and inward.

By high school, I was also playing vibes (a keyboard percussion instrument resembling the xylophone). I spent my high school summers playing at hotels in the Catskill Mountains resort area. These were "swinger" hotels. (Don't ask.) We played dance music during the week, and we backed up strippers and comedians on the weekends.

When we played the shows, I mainly watched the strippers, but I slumped down to play the vibes.

Whether I was playing or not, I was in the habit of slumping. I would slump down to play the vibes, collapse down to play the trumpet, and curve over to read a book. I lived in a slump.

Years later, I was playing vibes at a brunch gig, when I felt some pain in my right thumb. I figured it was nothing to worry about, and it would go away in a few days. But the pain got progressively worse, and it didn't take long for my whole hand to feel painful, weak, swollen, and tingly. I couldn't hold a toothbrush, a razor, my mallets, or a conversation.

My doctor prescribed anti-inflammatory and pain medications. She said to take them for a week or two and, if the pain persisted, make an appointment with a hand surgeon. I did, it did, so I did.

The earliest appointment for the surgeon was still a few months away. In the interim, I saw three chiropractors, two massage therapists, two acupuncturists, two Rolfers, one acupressurist, one Hellerworker, and a partridge in a pear tree.

The doctor won't see you now

When my appointment date finally arrived, I went to the office of what turned out to be hand specialist number one. He looked at a live x-ray of my hand and said, "Your hand is fine." My hand wasn't fine.

Specialist number two asked me if I ever had an MRI on my neck. I remember thinking, "What does my neck have to do with my hand?" As it turns out: everything. He had found a source of my pain.

The MRI revealed osteophytes (bone spurs) in my neck. The bone spurs were impinging on the nerves that ran down from my neck to my hand.

In addition to my hand pain (which was a pain in the neck), I was starting to get a pain in my neck (which was a pain in the ass).

The neck pain was debilitating. I couldn't take a step without experiencing a whole-body electric jolt. I thought this pain might last forever, which inspired a pain of its own.

My neck and hand pain had been so bad for so long that I met with a surgeon who specialized in the cervical spine. The surgeon told me he could fix me and demonstrated what the operation would entail, using a pen (substituting for a scalpel), and a skeleton (substituting for me).

But when he accidentally dropped his "scalpel" during the imaginary surgery, I decided to keep the surgery imaginary.

Luckily, I knew Phillip.

A new hope

Phillip, a sax-playing bandmate of mine, suggested I try the Alexander Technique (AT). He told me that his friend was scheduled for back surgery, took one single AT lesson, and was completely cured. This sounded too good to be true (and, as it turns out, it was too good to be true). But I gave the Alexander Technique a try and loved it from the start. For the first time in a long time I felt hope. I had been searching for someone to fix my neck and, at this very first lesson, I realized that I was that someone. If I could learn to live with less neck tension, my neck would have a chance to heal.

INTRODUCTION

F.M. Alexander (1869 – 1955) was an actor who was losing his voice during performances. After years of self-study, he realized his problem was stemming from his unconscious habit of gripping and clenching from head to toe.

Alexander came up with ways to loosen his grip and, in doing so, resolved his vocal issues. Little did he know that, in solving his problem, he was founding a new modality.

If you ask three Alexander Technique practitioners what the Alexander Technique is, you'll get five different answers. It has been described as a tension-relieving, posture-improving, awareness-raising, consciousness-expanding modality, but you can also use it while bowling. I used it for neck pain. I started studying AT in the late 1990s and was Certified by the American Center for the Alexander Technique (ACAT) teacher training program in 2003.

Learning AT helps you sit, stand, and walk with more ease. You release muscles you didn't know you were clenching, and thoughts you hadn't noticed you were gripping. Your posture will noticeably improve and your movements will be more fluid, but AT offers life-changing benefits and empowers you in unexpected ways.

This book is for those who are new to AT, as well as experienced practitioners and Alexander teachers. It includes 29 stories, jokes, and lessons. My intention is to present AT in a way that is light-hearted, practical, and immediately usable.

"Lighten UP" is my first book. The next one will also take 73 years, and it will be even shorter.

We had better get started.

1.

Pain in the neck

slumped into my first Alexander Technique lesson and plopped onto the stool opposite my teacher. After sitting on this stool for forty-five seconds, I asked for a chair with a back, because mine hurt—my back hurt, my neck hurt, and my shoulders had no idea where to go. Nothing was comfortable, and I was miserable.

I slumped out of that session with the same pain I had slumped in with, but I had a different mindset. I now knew there was a logical way to diminish and lose my neck pain.

It was at this lesson that I first heard the phrase: "free your neck." With familiarity and practice, those three little words can empower you.

Lesson: Free your neck

You free your neck muscles the same way you free other muscles—you release them, loosen them, un-tighten them, relax them, let them go.

Let's play with this idea.

Make a tight fist. Now turn your tight fist into a looser fist.

With your intention, you have freed your hand, finger, and forearm muscles. You may not know the name or function of every muscle, tendon, and nerve involved, and you may not know the exact science of how a thought translates into physical action. Yet, you easily freed the grip of your hand with a thought. In the same way, you can learn to release the habitual gripping of your neck muscles.

Now, cup your hands around your ears and hold your head firmly (please don't hurt yourself). Try to turn your head left and right, but prevent it from moving. You are tightening your neck muscles.

Remove your hands and allow your head to move easily. You have freed your neck.

As you practice freeing your neck, you'll notice that your nose may slightly lower while the crown of your head moves up. It's as if your head is rotating forward, and moving up, all because you're letting go of the muscles in your neck that tend to bring it down.

You don't need your hands to practice freeing your neck. You can free your neck any time you think of it.

You can free your neck right now.

2.

Of round-shouldered mice and me

During teacher training, I was living in a very small apartment in Queens. It was so small, the mice walked around round-shouldered. It was so small, you'd put the key in the door and you'd break the mirror. It was so small, you'd have to go out to the hall to change your mind.

I walked around the apartment somewhat round-shouldered *mice-self*, but not because the apartment was so small. My long-standing habit of slouching was still with me.

My shoulders were draping my collapsed rib cage. They found their resting place forward, down, and narrowed. But now, at least, I had a strategy. I knew the steps to un-round my shoulders, naturally.

Lesson: Unrounding your shoulders

Just as you released your fist in lesson one, release the muscles in your neck. (Remember, this may take a bit of practice.)

Freeing your neck will let your head rotate forward and move up.

Your head takes your spinal column up too.

Your rib cage, which is attached to your spinal column, moves upwards and outwards as well.

Your shoulders are poised on a rib cage that is no longer collapsed forward and down, so they are resting further back, and they're wider—naturally.

3.

Sit happens

In the AT world, we spend a good deal of time practicing "chairwork." Chairwork refers to sitting and standing with awareness, inhibition, and direction (more on that later). Chairwork covers so much. It includes the act of sitting down, the act of standing up, and all the things we do while seated or standing. It encompasses hinging forward to slurp your minestrone and squatting down to pet your dog. Chairwork deals with everything from soup to mutts.

Lesson: Sitting and standing

Standing up

If you are so inclined, stand up and then sit back down.

Stand up once more, but this time, notice if you're leading with your neck, poking it forward even before you leave the chair. You may also notice your chin raise. These are signs that you are preparing for standing by tensing.

Instead, before standing, free your neck to let your head move up. Let your sit bones release down into the chair. (The sit bones are the two "U" shaped bones at the bottom of your bottom.)

Practice freeing your neck while inclining forward and backward using your hip joints as hinges. Note that the hip joint hinges are lower than you might imagine. They are near the crease where your legs meet your torso (inches lower than the spot where you place your fingers when you put your hands on your "hips").

As your torso angles forward from your hip joints, let your gaze track down the wall in front of you. This will help you leave your neck alone.

Now, move your feet back a bit and walk your sit bones towards the front edge of the chair. If your heels come off the ground a bit, it's ok.

Hinge forward again, and when your weight is sufficiently over your feet, send your heels down into the floor. Your head moves up and you rise.

Sitting down

Feel for the front of the chair with the back of your legs.

Then, remember three important steps:

> *1. Your knees move forward*
>
> *2. Your hip joints move back*
>
> *3. We don't really need #3*

Bend your knees and hinge forward from your hip joints. Let your gaze move downward so that your neck isn't unnecessarily involved. Stay hinged forward from the hip joints until your legs and bottom reach the chair.

Then, think of your neck, head, and torso as one free, flexible unit, and hip-joint hinge back to neutral.

Your lower back softens, letting your sit bones release down into the seat.

4.

Bending down without ending down

Early on in our AT teacher training, we learned and practiced an athletic stance. Picture an infielder watching the batter, and you're envisioning an athletic stance. A batter watching the pitcher is also in an athletic stance. A tennis player waiting for the serve is using an athletic stance. But the athletic stance isn't just for athletes.

Parents can use it as they lower themselves towards their children. Children already use it as they lower themselves towards their toys. Percussionists can use it as they lower themselves towards their marimba. Alexander Technique teachers can use it as we lower our salary expectations.

This "mechanically advantageous" stance can be your dish-washing stance, coffee-making stance, and make-up stance. It's perfect for a jerky bus or a lurching train—good for brushing your teeth and your tennis game.

When you move towards an athletic stance, you are lowering yourself without shortening yourself. Your knees move forward and your hip joints move back, and that's it.

This stance hinges on your hinges. When you maximize the hinging while you minimize the bending you will give your neck a rest.

Lesson: The athletic stance

While standing, bend your knees.

Did you lean back? If so, your hip joints are going forward. For an athletic stance, you want your knees going forward but your hip joints going back.

Bend your knees again, but this time think: "knees forward, hip joints back."

This will put you in a free, flexible, athletic stance.

Remember the three steps of the athletic stance:

1. Knees forward

2. Hip joints back

3. That's pretty much it

5.

Below "see" level

Straight ahead or down is mostly where we're looking, because that's where stuff is. Our phone, our soup, the sidewalk with the dog poop—everything and the kitchen sink is at, or below, "see" level. Thankfully, most of the weight of the head is in front of the spine, so it's easy to rotate our head forward to look down.

Yes, we occasionally need to rotate our head backwards to look up at skies, clouds, ceilings, stars, and birds. It rotates backwards when we instill eye drops or gargle. It's what we do when we're on our bike, looking up the road. Our head rotates backward to get the first bite of pizza or the last drop of water.

But, most of the time
when we're walking around,
we're either looking straight ahead
or else we're looking down.

We watch where we're walking
which works out fine,
'cause most of our head's weight's
in front of our spine.

Lesson: Looking down and up

Put your index fingers in your ears and imagine that they are touching. You are pointing towards your atlanto-occipital (AO) joints. These joints are a natural hinging place from which to <u>rotate</u> your head forward to look down, and backward to look up.

As you look down and up, with your fingers still in your ears, notice that your fingers aren't lowering (as long as you're not collapsing). When you use your atlanto-occipital joints, you're looking down without collapsing down, and you're looking up without collapsing down

When reading, you can start looking down at your book, your phone, or your alphabet soup by using your eyes only. Then, let your head rotate forward using your AO joints. Your nose lowers but the crown of your head needn't.

[<u>Note</u>: To further reduce the reading angle, you can prop up your phone or book on a table. Bags, briefcases, and backpacks make great book, phone, and tablet holders on planes, trains, and automobiles.]

6.

Like riding a bike

Here I was, waking up at the crack of noon to go on my first bike ride post graduation. I was looking forward to riding again—getting out of the city, being on an open country road with the wind rustling through where my hair used to be.

As much as I wanted to forget everything and enjoy the ride, I had to keep my neck in mind to avoid pain. To that end, I freed my neck frequently and let my head tip forward and move up and away from my cervical spine.

Since I needed to angle my body forward to reach the handlebars and also look up to see the road, I hinged using the hip joint/AO joint combination.

The ride was great, but now I was ravenous. I headed home, cooked some food, and ate.

Eating has its challenges, especially if you have neck or back pain. If you slump down to the food, your neck and back muscles engage, in order to stop your face from becoming an ingredient. If you "sit up straight," your meal ends up on your shirt.

So, even while eating, I chose to pay attention to freeing my neck and using my hip joints.

Biking and eating both require the hip joint/AO joint combo. With practice, it comes naturally – like riding a bike.

Lesson: Hinging

For Biking

Find the freedom in your neck to let your head go where it yearns to go—tipping forward and moving up.

What's up? It's useful to think of "up" as your head moving away from whichever way your spine is pointed. When standing, up is straight up. When lying down, up is towards the wall behind you. When riding a bike, up is on a forward diagonal.

Reach for the handlebars, without slumping or tensing, by freeing your neck and hinging with your hip joints.

Because of the forward angle of your torso, you'll need to rotate your head back in order to see up the road. Use the hip/AO joint combination to let your head rotate backwards, easing up and away from the top of your spine.

For Eating

To get your mouth over the plate or bowl, again, hinge with your hip joints.

When you tip your torso forward using your hip joints, your mouth just goes along for the ride. You can always move back in your seat and hinge a little lower, should you want to get your mouth a little closer.

Use the hip/AO joint combo to tilt your head back but up—up and away from the top of your spine.

Take a moment and enjoy your meal.

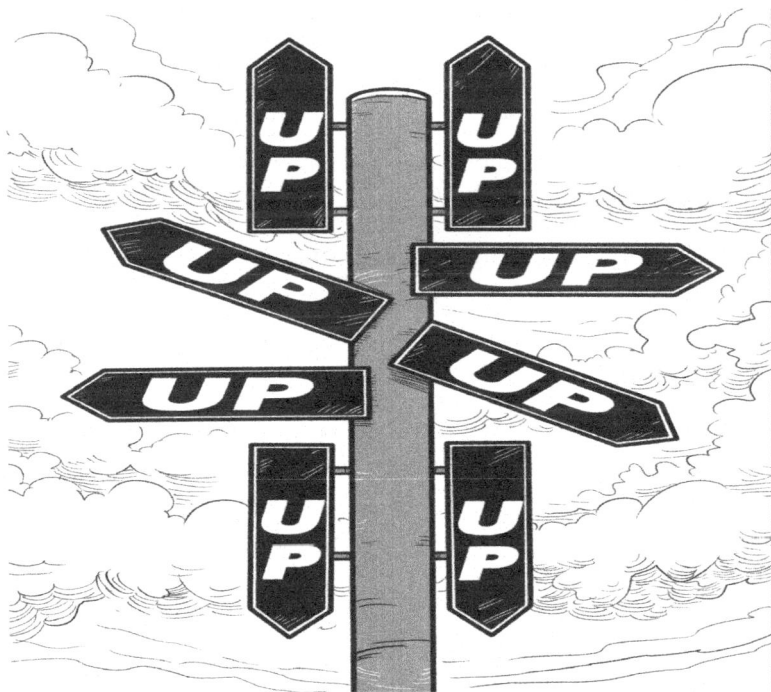

7.

Fight, flight, or bite

We tighten our jaw when we're stressed or obsessed. We tighten it when we're jealous, fearful, or angry. We clench our teeth when we tightly grip our viewpoints. Jaw-tightening can become a daily habit and teeth-grinding a nightly one. A dentist may give us a night guard, but that just guards our teeth at night. Our teeth get protected, but the tension continues, and the grinding grinds on.

The good news is: at any moment, you can stop to free your neck and jaw. It only takes seconds and it becomes a habit. The freer your jaw is in the daytime, when you're awake, the freer it could be at night, when you're not.

Lesson: Free your jaw

Free your neck and let go of your chewing muscles.

Let your lips lightly touch while your teeth are apart.

Think "ahhh" on a few in-breaths and out-breaths. Your throat is opening and your jaw is releasing.

Check to see if your tongue is pressing on the roof of your mouth or against your front teeth. If it is, let it release and air will take its place.

Open your mouth by letting your jaw move away and down from your top teeth. Notice if your head is rotating backwards—it doesn't have to.

With your mouth still open, free your chewing muscles once more.

Then, slowly let your lips come together until they are lightly touching—lips together, teeth apart. Breathe silently through your nose and lightly smile.

8.

Let's (not) grab a drink

We need extra tension like a moose needs a hatrack. Yet, we add it to all the things we do and all the thoughts we think.

We add tension when we sit, stand, and walk. We add it when we eat, shave, and drink. We clutch when we lift our beer glasses and clench when we remove our sunglasses. We overgrasp our cups and mugs when we're drinking and our phones and combs when we're not. We tense as we reach, and we grip when we get there.

Fortunately, all this gripping and grabbing is merely a habit, and habits can be broken.

Lesson: Drinking with ease

Find the freedom in your neck, ungrip your jaw, and let your head move up.

Your fingers will find your cup. Your torso can stay back and up. Use your hip joints, if you need them, to get closer.

Gently shape your hand when you get nearer to the cup. If you form the shape early, you may over-grasp.

Gently hold the cup with only the effort that is needed. Think of the cup as an extension of your fingertips, and let your fingertips lead as you bring your drink all the way up to your mouth—your mouth can stay back where it is.

When the cup reaches your lips, rotate your wrist to tilt it. Your jaw is free to open and move away from your face, as needed. Your head is free to tilt back, but up, if needed.

Lower the drink by moving your fingertips away from your mouth, towards the table. When your drink gently lands, expand your hand.

9.

Necknames

Left to our own devices, our devices own us. They suck us in, and they draw us down. We bow to them, and they shape us.

When we habitually stick our neck forward towards an object or a thought, it gets a neckname; like text neck, computer neck, fear neck, and future neck.

"Necks" are nothing new. We've had cave painting neck, hunting neck, tablet neck, and quill pen neck. Now we have tech neck, phone neck, keyboard neck, and tablet neck (again). Soon we'll have the next neck because it has never been the device or the thought; it has always been our reaction. The object or thought keeps changing, but the tendency to grasp it remains the same.

Lesson: Using devices

We automatically grip our devices with our eyes, and our eyes drag our neck forward.

To start breaking the gripping habit, forget about the device for just a moment.

Free your neck and let it ease back and up.

Your head will tip forward and move up, as if on its own.

You can get your eyes closer to your device by moving the device, or by using your hip joints.

Let your neck be free, uncommitted, back, and up.

It's not like your neck doesn't care, it's just that it isn't involved. And when your neck isn't involved, it won't get a neckname.

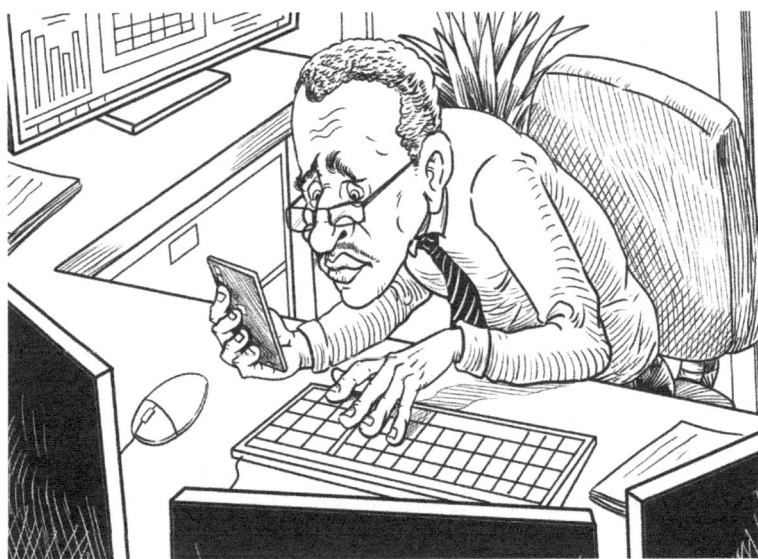

10.

Take ten

On my way to teaching in Manhattan, I had time to go to "World's Best Coffee," which has the third best coffee on the block. I order my coffee with "no sugar, please" which is always an adventure. "No sugar, please" needs to be accompanied by hand signals, head shaking, and side-to-side finger-wagging... and it still doesn't work.

Baristas have the deeply-ingrained habit of adding sugar to coffee. As soon as they hear "coffee," they reach for the spoon to dip in the sugar, and they dream about their weekend while they're filling up the cup.

Likewise, we have deeply-ingrained habits with our devices. As soon as we sit at the computer, we grip with our eyes as we stick our face forward, and we tighten our jaw as we grab for the mouse.

Sitting all crunched and tensed like this is hard on our joints, hard on our spine, hard on our posture, and hard on our mind.

"Take frequent breaks" is the advice we usually hear, but after we take a break from our device, we often don't go back to neutral—we go back to our habits.

Lesson: Computer break

Gently take your hands off the keyboard for a moment, and let them rest by your sides.

Place your attention on the back of your neck and let go of some tension there. Add the intention, as you loosen those muscles, that your head will tip forward and move up on its own.

Let your lower back release, and your sit bones find the seat. You're going up and down. You're lengthening yourself.

With your arms still by your sides, move your hand a few inches forward toward the keyboard. Do it once more, this time thinking of leading with your fingertips. (Your hand doesn't need to change its shape.) When thinking of your fingertips doing the leading, your elbow bends without shortening, and your arm freely moves without tightening.

Wait until your fingers are near the keyboard to shape your hand, avoiding "endgaining" (rushing towards a goal).

Your jaw is free, your breathing is easy, and your shoulders are poised on your ribcage.

Think of the opposition between your head and your sit bones.

Think of the opposition between your eyes and your computer.

Free your neck, slightly smile, and fully breathe.

11.

Resting on the Hudson

Neck discomfort was still a factor while I was a tuxedoed musician on World Yacht, a dinner cruise ship. We circled around the southern tip of Manhattan playing music for dinner and dancing, six nights per week, for years.

During some of that time, I had to go up to the boat's wheelhouse and do "constructive rest." And I mean *had* to. Standing hurt my neck and so did sitting. The next best choice was lying down.

I would do constructive rest in the ship's filthy wheelhouse. The wheelhouse is the crew's room. The cruise's crews' shoes were covered in crud. The crud was a mixture of sewer sludge, filet mignon drippings, boot-smashed potatoes, diesel fuel, and cake. This cruddy rug was the rug I would lie on in my tux.

I'd lie on my back, my head resting on a few paperback books. Having my head fully supported, while freeing my neck, gave me an instant wave of relief. My spine was no longer weight-bearing, which helped me lengthen and widen.

My knees were bent and my feet were on the grimy floor. I repeatedly released my neck and my jaw. I let my entire torso move with my breathing, and I was breathing as if I were out of pain.

Then it was time to go down to the main floor and play. But I couldn't just yank myself up off the floor (and not just because I was sticking to it). I had to think about *how* to get up from the floor, so as not to undo the good that I'd done.

I freed my neck first. My gaze moved to the side, my head followed, then my torso. From hands and knees, I came all the way up and walked taller to the bandstand.

Lesson: Constructive rest

When you have a bit of time, lie on the floor facing up. If you need assistance getting down to the floor, find a person or a piece of furniture to help you out. Let go of any grip on your neck on your downward journey.

Use something to prop up your head. Paperback books are best, but if they're not available, use a backpack, a jacket, or a towel— whatever's around. You don't want the books too high or too low. Look for a little forward tip of your head.

Your hands can rest by your sides or on your stomach, whatever suits you.

Your knees are bent with your feet on the floor.

Let the floor completely take your weight.

De-tense any tensing and unclench any clenching. There's nothing to grasp at, not even a thought.

Watch as your head, arms, and legs move away from your torso— not because you're moving them, but because you're ungripping them and adding that intention.

When it's time to get up, look to the side, because that's the way you'll roll. Your eyes will lead your head, and your head will lead your torso.

Help yourself to your hands and knees.

You might plant one foot, free your neck, and rise all the way up to your newer, truer, taller stature.

12.

The whispered oy

A Texas rancher and a New York Rabbi sat next to each other on a train. The Texan bragged about how much bigger everything is in Texas. He said that his property was so large that he could start driving at seven in the morning and wouldn't reach the end of his property till six at night!

The Rabbi responded, "Yeah, I had a car like that once."

I had a car like that too. My van went from zero to sixty in three weeks. But it got me to gigs, and it got me out of the city and into nature. I would leave crowded, busy Manhattan and get into the woods in an hour.

As soon as I got out of the car, I would feel more peaceful.

My breathing would slow down and deepen. My facial muscles would let go. My neck seemed to free, as if on its own. Hearing the leaves rustling in the wind was like hearing nature whisper "ah" and it made me want to "ah" along.

Lesson: Alexander's Whispered Ah

Think of the woods, a person, a place, a pet, a flower, a joke, or anything that will make you genuinely smile. The smile may start in the corners of your eyes, and spread to the corners of your mouth.

Open your mouth by letting your jaw move away and down. Exhale slowly and fully, whispering "ahhh"—not spoken, only whispered.

Then, with your lips lightly touching, let the air come in through your nose, silently. Your whole torso expands.

When you are comfortably full, free your jaw and let it move away and down, whispering "ahhh" again.

Take your time

Let the lips come together and let the air back in.

Whisper one more wide-open, easy "ahhh."

Notice the calm.

13.

IKEA:
"We put the ouch in couch"

I live across the street from a hospital, which is convenient because I sometimes buy furniture from IKEA. You take IKEA furniture home in parts and attempt to put it together. When you notice that there is a piece missing and the directions are blank, frustration sets in. You may rush to get the job over with and "endgain."

One day, in the over-focused, neck-tensing, endgaining rush to finish my couch, I cut my finger. I walked across the street to the hospital, and found the IKEA ward by following the arrows and sniffing for meatballs.

As I was assembling my waiting room chair, they called my name. I was bandaged and sent home.

All's well that ends well, but things would have ended better had I inhibited my tendency to endgain. Endgaining never helps, often hurts, and can even cut a finger.

Lesson: What is endgaining?

Endgaining is overemphasizing the result and underemphasizing the process. It's rushing towards a finish line in a state of tension. Endgaining is obsessively fixating on an outcome. It's getting ahead of yourself.

When we endgain, we're intensely concentrating on the what, while being inattentive to the how. There's too much then and not enough now. Our mind is in the future and our neck is presently tensed.

Endgaining is watching the flight of a golf ball that hasn't yet flown. Endgaining pokes our neck forward as we start to stand up. Endgaining is a clenched jaw, gripped hands, and a tight, graspy mind.

But once you're aware that you're endgaining, you can stop it right in its tracks. You can pause, free your neck, and redirect. You can let your endgaining, future-living, forward-thrusting neck come back and up to the freedom of the present.

Keep the goals, lose the grasping. Keep the love, lose the grip. Respond instead of merely reacting. Stay back and mind the gap.

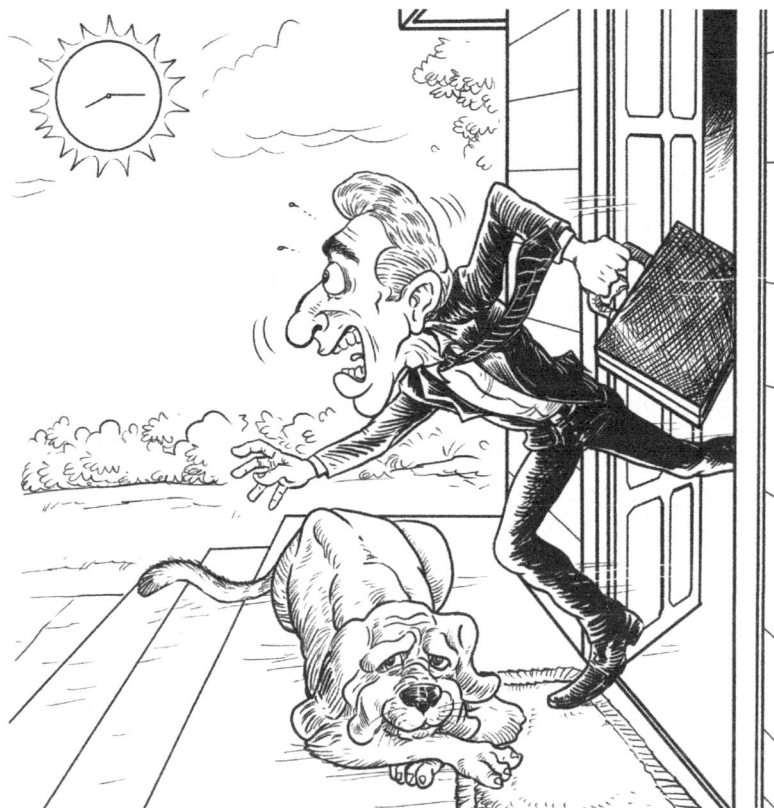

14.

Mind the gap

As it is commonly used, the word "inhibition" has negative connotations. It tends to be understood as something restricting—something tight, limiting, and confining.

Alexander's inhibition is different.

Alexander's inhibition is a non-reactive space that you can create anytime. This gap provides an alternative to mindlessly rushing ahead or aimlessly traveling down the well-worn rut of habit. Inhibition is a clearing, and from that clearing, your direction flows.

Viktor E. Frankl's ideas in *Man's Search for Meaning* have been summarized: "Between stimulus and response there is a space. In that space is our power to choose our response. In our response lies our growth and our freedom."

Watch as baseball players inhibit as they refuse to swing at an outside pitch, and hear guitarists inhibit as they leave space for the music to breathe.

Teachers inhibit, comedians inhibit... sculptors exhibit, and frogs inribbit.

Cats pause for the cause with their claws, as all four of their paws pause—'cause cats wait for the right moment to pounce. Cats inhibit.

You can use inhibition when you notice you're worrying, reacting to something that isn't even happening and may never happen.

At any moment, you can become aware, create a gap, free your neck, and change direction. You can apply inhibition to washing dishes, playing bassoon, or bowling.

Lesson: Applying inhibition

Washing dishes

Pause and free your neck.

Freely move towards an athletic stance. The lower the sink, the deeper the angle.

Pause before reaching for a dish. Think of leading more with your fingertips, less with your neck.

Resist shaping your hand around the dish until the last moment. Then hold it with only the effort that is needed, inhibiting the habit of grasping.

Inhibit again before you reach for the dish soap. Use more aware-ness and less tension than is your habit.

If you have an extra minute and are so inclined, you may want to put the dish down and start from the top.

Playing bassoon

Leave a gap before you reach for your bassoon case, then reach for it with minimal effort.

If you are unnecessarily raising your shoulder when you're reaching—smile, let it lower, wait a sec, and do it over.

Inhibit before every new movement phrase of unpacking, assembling, and playing.

Bowling

Way, way before thinking about the pins, the beer, and the pizza— leave some space, free your neck, and notice your breathing.

On an outbreath, do a Whispered Ah. If the bowling alley is crowded, feel no pressure to open your mouth widely.

Do several more inconspicuous Whispered Ahs.

Allow your neck, arms, and shoulders to be as free as possible, even while holding and swinging the weight of the ball.

Come back and up to the present moment, and bowl here now.

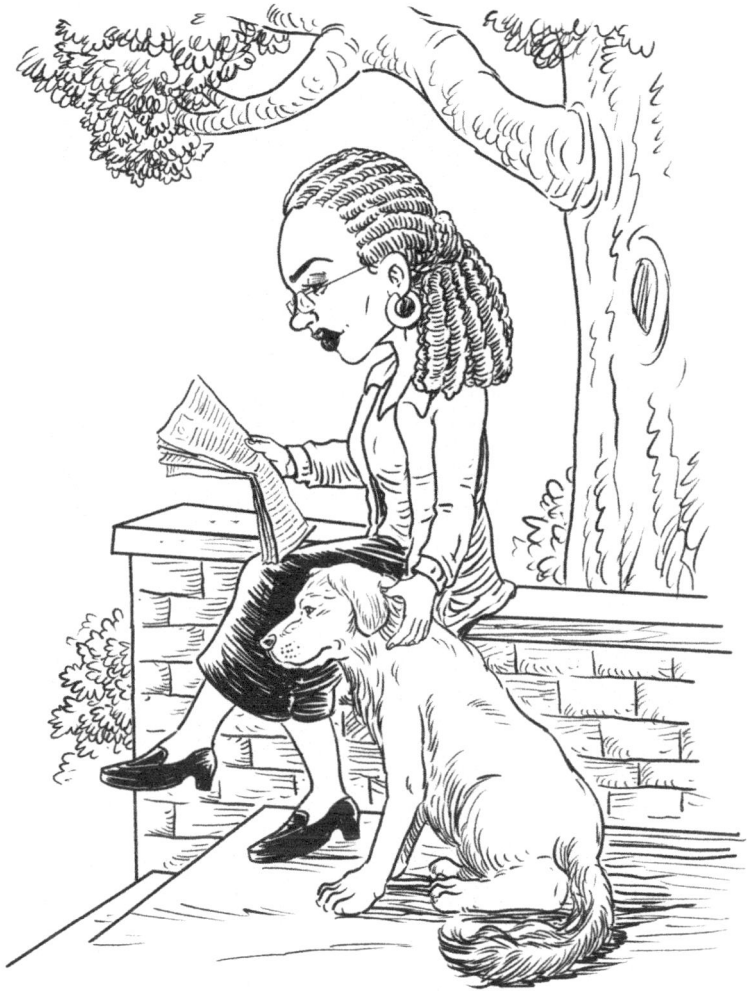

15.

To don't list

There are Alexander directions you may apply to specific actions and primary directions you apply to anything at all.

The primary directions are primarily preventative. They form more of a "to don't" list than a "to do" list. There is more undoing than doing—more subtraction than addition.

The primary directions sometimes read:

> *I wish to free my neck so that*
> *my head can move forward and up,*
> *so that my torso can lengthen and widen,*
> *and my legs can move away from my torso,*
> *and my shoulders release out the sides.*

Lesson: The primary directions

When considering the primary directions, look for the subtextual "to don't" list embedded within it.

"I wish to free my neck so that my head can move forward and up."

> *Don't tighten your neck and pull your head back and down.*

"So that my torso can lengthen and widen."

> *Don't shorten and narrow your torso.*

"And my legs can move away from my torso."

> *Don't grip the muscles surrounding your hip joints.*

"And my shoulders release out the sides."

> *Don't let your shoulders drape forward and down and don't pull them back "military posture" style.*

16.

Slump life

About twenty-five AT teacher-trainees were sitting in a semicircle facing the teacher, who was sitting in an uncharacteristic, exaggerated slump.

The teacher asked, "What is wrong with the way I'm sitting?"

Each trainee was asked to express one idea. They called out their suggestions:

> "Your torso is being shortened.''
>
> "Your breathing is compromised."
>
> "You're pulling down."

When everyone had their say, she responded, "There's nothing wrong with the way I'm sitting..."

As she transformed out of her slump, she continued, "...unless I live there."

Weeks later, I got a call from my doctor. He had some not-so-great news about a recent lab result. He told me to come in as soon as possible to repeat the test.

I immediately slumped with my arm against a wall. But unlike my habitual slump, this slump was done on purpose, consciously. It was as if, at that moment, I wanted my physical state to reflect my mental state.

After a short while, I came out of the slump and decided that I would deal with everything later. I chose not to live in a bad news slump. (Spoiler alert: everything was fine.)

Lesson: Don't live in a slump

As soon as you become aware that you're slumping, inhibit the quick fix of immediately sitting up straight.

Instead, free your neck, and let your head rise.

When your head rises, you rise. You're sitting taller, your breathing is easy, and your mood might be lighter too.

When you find yourself slumping again, don't worry. Moment by moment, time after time, you can easefully come out of your slump. Slump if you want, just don't live there.

17.

Slumpacino Grande

I was in the mood to pay too much money for a cup of coffee, so I headed for Starbucks. I tipped the maitre d to get my own small table, "non-sticky, extra dry please."

While wrestling with the folded-up napkin and table leg, I was greeted by that familiar aroma trifecta: burnt coffee, rancid cinnamon, and the bathroom.

I glanced over at a tall young woman at the next table who was stooped over her laptop and her Tall Caramel Mocha Frappuccino with unsweetened soy milk.

The table was too low, or the stool too high, and she adapted by adopting a downward "c" curve towards her coffee, computer, and cookie. The coffee was a Tall, but she was sitting small—she was in the Starbucks Slump and we've all *bean* there.

Lesson: Coming out of a slump

The most important part of coming out of a slump is the moment you become aware that you're in a slump.

The very next step is not berating yourself for being in a slump.

Then, take a second to let go of the idea of posture, posturing, posing, or positions. Forget "stomach in, chest out, shoulders back, and tuck your chin." Erase the tension-filled picture of "a string pulling your head up."

Instead, look for some freedom in your neck.

Your freeing neck lets your head tip forward and move up, leading your spine up.

Your sit bones release down to the chair, creating a peaceful opposition to your neck, head, and torso that are rising. You're easefully sitting taller, your neck is not poking forward, you're out of your slump, and your breathing is fuller.

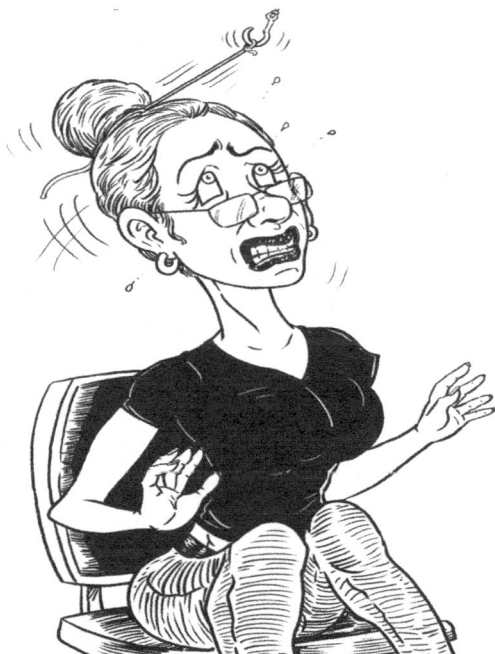

18.

Tooth haste

We brush our teeth on autopilot. We unthinkingly tense our neck, grasp our hands, grab the brush, and tighten our shoulders. We poke our neck forward and down, and our head rotates back and down.

But, if we take a moment to inhibit, free our neck, and let our head rise, we can brush our teeth with ease.

Here's more, in an Alexander Technique-infused toothbrushing poem.

Lesson: Toothbrushing

We poke our neck forward to get our teeth to the brush,
instead of the other way around.
Our neck tightens, our shoulders raise
and our head rotates back and down.

Then we grasp the brush as if it weighed a ton
and someone's going to rip it from our grip.
We jam the brush to our teeth, much harder than we need
and hurt our lip, our tooth could chip, our spit may drip.

Instead, gently hold the brush and bring it up to your teeth
using only the effort that is needed.
Brush your teeth gently, without tensing your elbow,
think that your fingertips are doing the leading.

Loosen up your neck and loosen it again
and watch your head as it raises from your spine.
Your knees are going forward and your hip joints going
back, and that's it—you're in a zig-zag kind of line.

When it's time to spit, you can lower your mouth
without putting pressure on your spine.
Let your knees go farther forward and your hip joints
farther back, it's a deeper, lower, zig-zagged line this time.

But we can brush all we want
and do it with ease,
we still may hear the drill and get the bill
and pay the fees of Dr. Feelbad.

19.

Doctor Feelbad

A trip to the dentist is like a bad marriage. It's expensive, it's painful, you don't get to talk, and people keep shoving metal tools in your mouth.

Will the Alexander Technique help you at the dentist? Of floss it will. And when drilling down, I would have to be numb or sedated not to extract that a dentist appointment would be deeply impacted by AT's crowning wisdom. At least that's what eye like tooth ink.

Lesson: AT at the dentist

Notice some neck freedom as you flip through the magazines. Let that freedom grow.

Think that your freeing neck muscles are cascading up and down your whole body.

Free your jaw and notice your breathing.

Your head moves up and your shoulders are poised on your ribcage.

Now you can better handle the soft yet somehow annoying music, the mournful whirring of the slow grinding drill, and the people screaming as they see their bill.

"Mark Ho..hofist...burke...joses...burd...jofes..."

Do some Whispered Ahs as they mispronounce your name.

You'll eventually be led out of the waiting room and into the treatment room. It's now time to climb onto that scary chair, albite reluctantly.

Ungrip your fingers, un-clench your jaw, and de-grip your toes.

Don't be a big shot—ask for a pillow if you need one.

Have your neck be as easy as possible throughout the entire ordeal, and don't think of it as an ordeal.

As you open your mouth, know that your head doesn't have to rotate back. Let your head incline forward and go up, away from the top of your spine.

Soften the muscles in the corners of your eyes. Soften the muscles in the corners of your mouth. Soften the muscles in your forehead.

Calm anxious thoughts by not following them - Follow your breath instead.

20.

Walk this way

A man walks over to a clerk in a drug store and asks for talcum powder. The clerk says, "Sure, walk this way."

After watching the clerk walk, the man says, "If I could walk that way, I wouldn't need the talcum powder."

Walk *what* way?

Naturally, rhythmically, easefully upright, and cat-like.

Cats lead with their heads, and their spine follows. We need to do the same, but we're upright. When our head leads our spine, it needs to lead it skyward. If we walk with a downward energy, it's hard on our body, joints, spine, and mind.

Lesson: Walking

Step one, in taking a step, is freeing your neck to let your head up.

When you take that first step, notice what moves forward first. Is it your chin? Your chest? Your foot?

Experiment with your knee moving forward first. (Though it doesn't need to be overly lifted.)

Let the heel touch the ground first, then the balls of the feet, then the toes. Heel, ball, toes...heel, ball, toes.

The rhythm is not even, though. It's more like

    Heel, b–a–l–l,   t—o—e—s.

    Heel, b–a–l–l,   t—o—e—s.

Let the toes of your back foot have their time on the ground. You'll get that cat-like roll-off, and get that cat-like roll-on.

When you free your neck when you're walking, your torso will naturally spiral—the right shoulder moves forward with the left knee, and the left shoulder moves forward with the right knee. Because your torso is spiraling, your arms will naturally swing.

21.

The museum walk

One of my students, Bob, had overcome lower back pain and was living symptom-free. But, after a museum visit, some pain returned. At first, he was confused. He had walked long distances before and his back was fine. What was the difference? Why the resurgence?

We realized that the pain recurred because of *how* he was walking in the museum. It wasn't his rhythmic, spiraling, upward-moving walk, and he wasn't walking at his normal pace.

Bob was doing the "museum walk." And we've all done it.

When we do the museum walk, we may take a few slow steps and stand, then a few more lazy steps and stand again. The walk becomes a heavy plod. Our torso gets drawn forward and down. Our neck, head, mood, and energy sinks. It takes more effort to shift weight, so we overplay the left-right sway.

Lesson: Walking slowly

Walking really slowly tends to draw us down, so in a museum, kitchen, or store, "mind the up."

You mind the up when you free your neck and let your head move up. And when you free your neck to let your head move up, your torso goes along for the ride. And when your neck, head, and torso move up, the museum walk and its exaggerated sway fades away.

To minimize the sway, maximize the up—keep the sway at bay by going up.

22.

Salmon says, "go up."

We need extra tension like a fish needs a bicycle, but that doesn't mean we should free our neck only to flop to the floor and flounder like a flounder. Free your neck for *shore*, but *up* is where we want to go, and going up takes intention and energy.

Lesson: Releasing without collapsing

If you free your neck and "do less" with no other consideration, you're not moving up, you're sinking down. So, free your neck, but have a strong intention to let your head float up to its natural, poised, newly heightened home.

If you notice some muscles (perhaps your abs) engaging on your way up—let them. Perhaps they were under-engaged. They are now engaging as a side effect, a bi-product of adding the intention to lengthen and bubble up.

While seated, let your sit bones anchor down in a friendly opposition to your head rising up.

Sole, as you perch on your chair, free your neck, but go up. Something's fishy with your phone bill? Free your neck and go up. Are you swimming in bills, oar drowning in debt? Free your neck and go up. Go up—You're not just freeing your neck for the halibut.

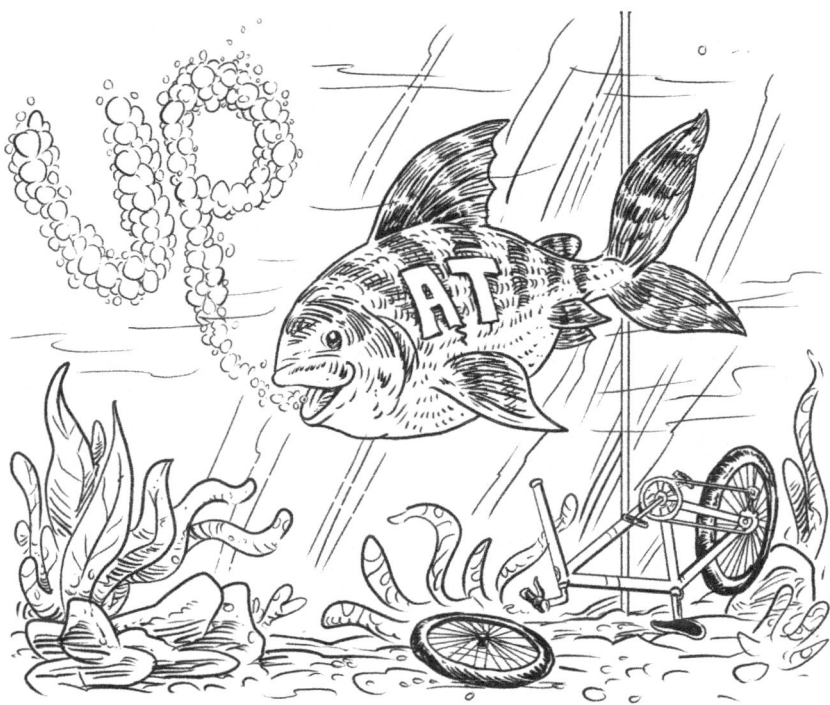

23.

Throb-o

I named my various neck and hand pains, hoping that I could cre-ate some space between the pain and myself. I also named them because I wanted to add a little lightness. In my case, there were three distinct pain sensations:

> 1. Hot'n Oily: A feeling of burning hot oil dripping down from my neck to my shoulders.

> 2. Palm Pain: A sensation as if I had used my palms to drive nails into concrete.

> 3. Tingly: It tingled.

When the pain flared up, I thought to myself: "hello, Hot'n Oily", or "well, here comes Tingly", or "welcome back, P.P." Naming my pain was just enough of a "joke" to help me take a step back.

Lesson: Name your pain

When pain pops up, we often react with a jolt and immediately tense up, which makes things worse. Instead, create distance between yourself and your pain, and become an observer. It may sound impossible, but you may even be able to find some humor.

If you want to give pain-naming a try, pay attention to the sensations in your body. What does it feel like? How would you describe it?

Achy, Jolty, Pulsie, Burnie, Stabby, Hipster, Needles, Knee-no, Anklet, Light-ning, and Pin-prick are some possible pain names. Use these or, even better, make up your own.

Whenever one of your "friends" arises, you can greet it. By adding distance, lightness, and Alexander directions, you'll be better able to respond to your pain by releasing, instead of reacting by tensing.

24.

Here Comes the Sun

When our neck is stiff and painful, we feel like we have to move our whole body just to turn our head. It's as if there is a block of ice around our neck. This block of ice serves as a self-imposed cast. With time you can learn to free your neck, melt that ice, and Let It Be.

Lesson: Melting tension

Imagine—The ice-brace is slowly melting and forming a pool of warm water. In that small area of warmer water, you can make slight, smooth, free head movements.

All Together Now, your neck thaws, your head softens upwards, your jaw defrosts, and your shoulders unfreeze.

Your ice-cast has liquified, your tension has vaporized, and a smile returns to your face.

All You Need Are Gloves.

25.

(Don't) sleep tight

Once in a while, I forget how to fall asleep. I turn off the lights, I get into bed, and then I lay there. I figure that closing my eyes is a good idea, so I close them. And I wait.

After a while, I realize nothing is happening. Then I remember to use some AT tools.

Lesson: Falling asleep

Free your neck as you get into bed or when you're already in bed. Avoid starting out in a compressed curve as you go to sleep or go back to sleep.

Experiment with starting on your back or your side.

While sleeping on your back, you can use a pillow under your knees if it suits you. Use a pillow under your head, allowing a slightly forward head rotation.

When sleeping on your side, use one pillow under your head, one between your knees, and one between your upper arm and torso.

Once you're comfortable, you may want to do some Whispered Ahs. The ease, depth, and rhythm of the Whispered Ah resembles our breathing pattern during sleep, helping to create a smooth transition from this world to the dreamworld.

Ease up your neck, un-clench your jaw, release your fingers, un-grasp your thoughts, and breathe.

26.

Walking, shaving, and eating a banana at the beach

The Alexander Technique is nothing if not practical. So, how do you walk, shave, and eat a banana at the beach without stubbing your toe or nicking your face? By walking softly and carrying a big schick.

Lesson: Walking, shaving, and eating a banana at the beach

Walking

As always, let go of your neck by letting go of any gripping there. Because you freed your neck, your head moves up with a slight forward tilt.

Your torso moves up, and one knee moves forward. Your heel touches the sand first, then the ball of the foot, then your toes. Heel, ball, toes.

Heel, b–a–l–l,   t–o–e–s.

Let the toes on the back foot have their time on the sand. When you smoothly roll-off, you can smoothly roll-on.

Shaving

Think that the handle of the razor is an extension of your fingertips. Mindfully move your fingertips, with the razor, to your face. Your fingertips are leading your arm; there's no need to raise your shoulder or tighten your elbow.

You might want to practice by bringing it back up to your face again, this time with even less tension.

Bananas

As you did with the razor, think of the banana as an extension of your fingertips. Bring the banana to your face—not your face to the banana. As the banana approaches, let your jaw move away and down. Take a piece gently, and don't bite off more than you can chew.

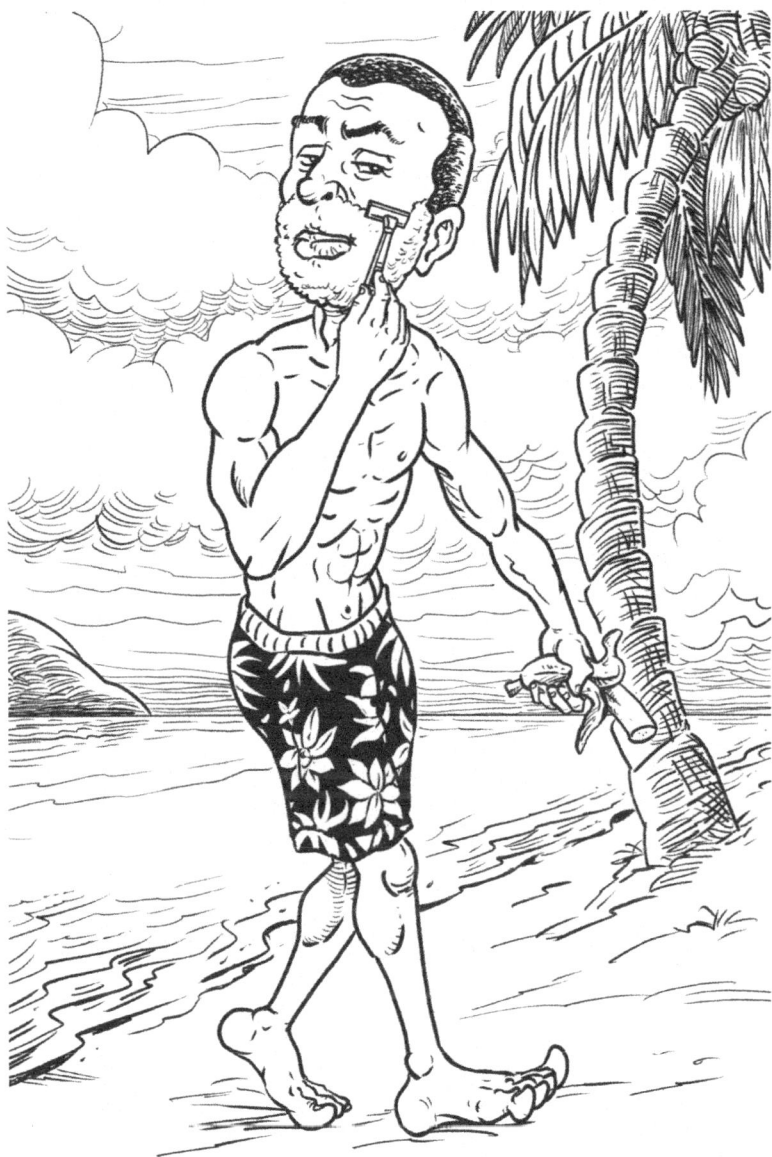

27.

Love and pain

AT teacher Elisabeth Walker said that her "use" (i.e. the way she used her body) was at its worst when she was knitting. She said: "I think it's because I *love* it so much."

It's love that draws us to our knitting, our book, the vanilla cake, and the chocolate mousse. Love draws us towards our music, sushi, and art.

Musical instruments call their musicians closer, and musicians surrender to the sound. Musicians dive in, neck first.

Sushi chefs sink to sushi's level as they corkscrew down to shape their fish.

Drawing draws the artist's eyes forward and down, and the neck goes where the eye is drawn.

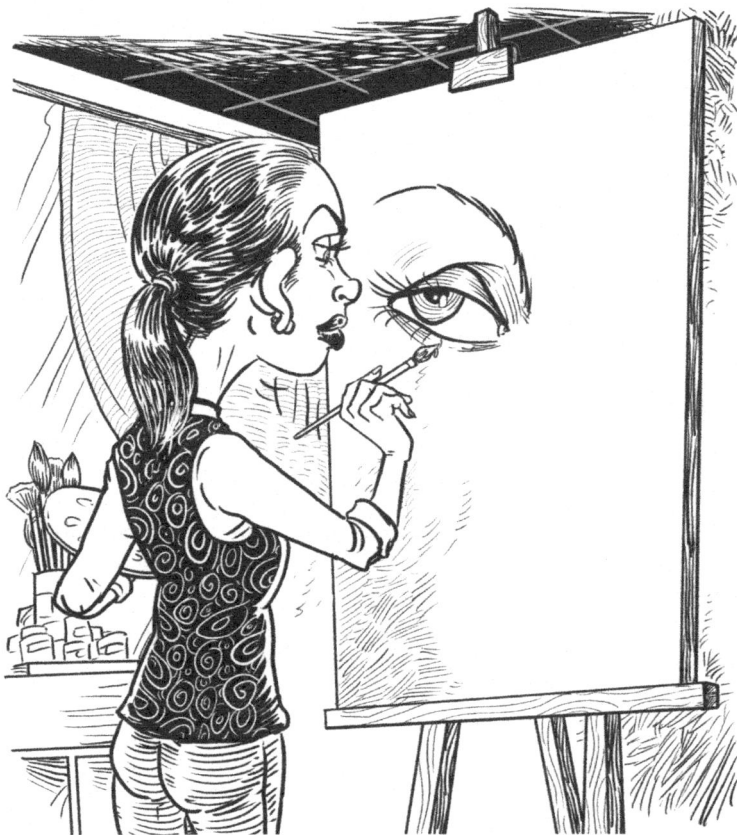

Lesson: Keep the love. Lose the grip.

Let go of the grip of the muscles in your neck and your head will move up on its own.

Free your neck again and watch as your nose lowers and your crown raises.

Let go of the grip in your lower back and your sit bones will release towards your chair.

Let your jaw dangle with your lips lightly touching.

Let your throat open up as if you're about to whisper "ahhh."

Your shoulders are poised; they're not needed right now.

Release the muscles around your hip joints and let your legs move away from your torso.

Think of something funny or pleasant and allow the faintest hint of a smile.

On an out-breath, whisper a wide-open "ahhh" as you release your jaw down and away.

The air silently comes in through your nose with your lips lightly touching.

Whisper a long, slow, controlled "ahhh" again.

Lips together teeth apart on a spacious in-breath.

Ah once more, doing less with your neck and watch as your head moves up.

Engage with what you love with mindfulness.

Keep the love. Lose the grip.

28.

Ouch. Ouch.

Falling asleep with chronic neck pain was a crapshoot. The pain would either prevent me from falling asleep altogether, or I would fall asleep and wake in an hour.

Thoughts raced around my mind: "Will this ever end? Is this the way it will be forever?"

This is the pain of the second arrow—the mind pain we add to the physical pain. Buddha said, "In life, we cannot always control the first arrow. However, the second arrow is our reaction to the first. And with this second arrow comes the possibility of choice."

Many years ago on a cold, rainy, miserable, painful evening, I burnt my forearm on a white-hot halogen light bulb. It hurt like hell, but as it turned out, it was just what I needed.

That night, like many other nights, I fell asleep but woke up in an hour. I immediately felt pain. But the main pain I was feeling was from my arm, not my neck. Unlike my neck pain, I knew that this new arm pain was temporary. I was aware of how and when this pain started, and I pretty much knew when it would end.

The new pain was a distraction from my chronic neck pain. It was almost a relief. I was able to fall back asleep with ease, because I had avoided the pain of the second arrow.

Lesson: The pain of the second arrow

When pain, whether physical or mental, comes to the foreground, inhibit identifying with it or grabbing at it. Instead, move your attention to your neck and let the tension melt away.

Let your jaw move down and away from your skull, and let your head move up and away.

Fully experience the sensation of your breathing. Listen attentively to the wide-open sound of a slow, easy, Whispered Ah. Listen for the silence of the inhalation.

Your attention has moved from any discomfort to the peaceful feeling that mindful breathing creates.

29.

Constructive Conscious Cultivation of the Individual

Have you ever found yourself feeling anxious, seemingly about nothing in particular? Have you ever found yourself obsessing or worrying about something small? Have you ever found yourself going round and round in circles of endless, repetitive thoughts?

The good news is: you've found yourself. You have become aware.

You can develop the skill of recognizing these kinds of triggering thoughts more quickly—before they have the chance to take hold, tensing your neck and restricting your breath. When needless worries no longer control your breathing, your body, or your attention, they fade away.

Lesson: Meditating

Stop for a second.

Put your attention on your neck freeing, your head rising, and the physical sensation of your breathing.

Take your time.

Your easing neck allows your head to rotate forward and move up. Your head leads your torso up, while you let your shoulders release, and your sit bones find the seat.

Soften the muscles surrounding your eyes and mouth.

If your breathing is shallow or if it's deep, it's correct.

Notice that the inbreath is cooler than the outbreath and stay with this sensation for a few minutes.

You can close your eyes.

You've got time.

Within seconds, random thoughts may appear, or your mind may have already latched onto a specific thought that whisked you away. Several minutes might have gone by before you even noticed.

Once you become aware of these thoughts, choose not to follow them, whether they are positive, negative, or neutral. Again and again, notice your thoughts and let them dissolve, as you shift your attention back to your breathing.

CONCLUSION

One final word about those three little words—"Free your neck."

"Neck" is a useful word, especially in a clothing store, but let's not limit it. To get as much power as you can from "free your neck," expand your idea of "neck." Let it mean more than just the area between your tee shirt collar and your jaw or head—more than just the place to hang your tie or scarf.

Your neck muscles start at your head and cascade down your back, shoulders, and chest. Some "neck muscles" go all the way down to your pelvis, so you're not just freeing your neck.

Why not further broaden the meaning of those three little words, so that when you free your neck, you also un-clench your jaw?

But it's even more than that.

Let "free your neck" wash over your whole self—mind, body, and spirit, giving you an instant wave of freedom, and relief.

You can free your neck right now.

When you free your neck to let your head up, notice how it changes your breathing.

Let "free your neck" calm you, and empower you.

RESOURCES

T hank you for reading.

I teach in-person lessons in NYC, as well as individual and group lessons online.

Visit MarkJosefsberg.com to schedule an online lesson and join my newsletter.

Email: Mark@MarkJosefsberg.com
to schedule an in-person lesson or ask a question.

American Society for the Alexander Technique (AmSAT)
AmSATonline.org

The Complete Guide to the Alexander Technique
AlexanderTechnique.com

THANK YOU

Steve, Peg, and the Josefsberg family

Alexis Martin

Susan and Alan Bowers, Michael Hanko

American Center for the Alexander Technique (ACAT) directors Joan Frost, Barbara Kent, Brooke Lieb

ACAT teachers:
Pearl Ausubel, Bob Bradley, Elizabeth Buonomo, Keisha Chin, Robert Cohen, Marta Curbelo, Joan Frost, Kim Jessor, Barbara Kent, Judith Lakin, Brooke Lieb, Hope Martin, Pat McGinness, Katherine Miranda, Cynthia Reynolds, Connie Serchuk, Loren Shlaes, Daniel Singer, Judy Stern, Dianne L. Sussman, Arthur Tobias Caren Bayer, Pedro DeAlcantara, Alex Farkas, Bruce Fertman, Michael Gelb, John Nicholls, Vivien Schapera, Marie Stroud, Elisabeth Walker, Lucia Walker, Nanette Walsh

ACAT classmates:
Bette Chamberlain, Ruth Diamond, Lisa Goldberg, Stephanie Kalka, Naoko Matsumoto

Martine Batchelor, Stephen Batchelor, Michael J. Gelb, Geshe Kelsang Gyatso, Clare Maxwell, Kadam Morten, Jessica Penzias, Robert Rickover, Rebecca Tuffey